CHRISTIANA BAYODE

At Home Workout for Busy Women

Easy Ways to Lose Weight and Tone up Without Going to the Gym

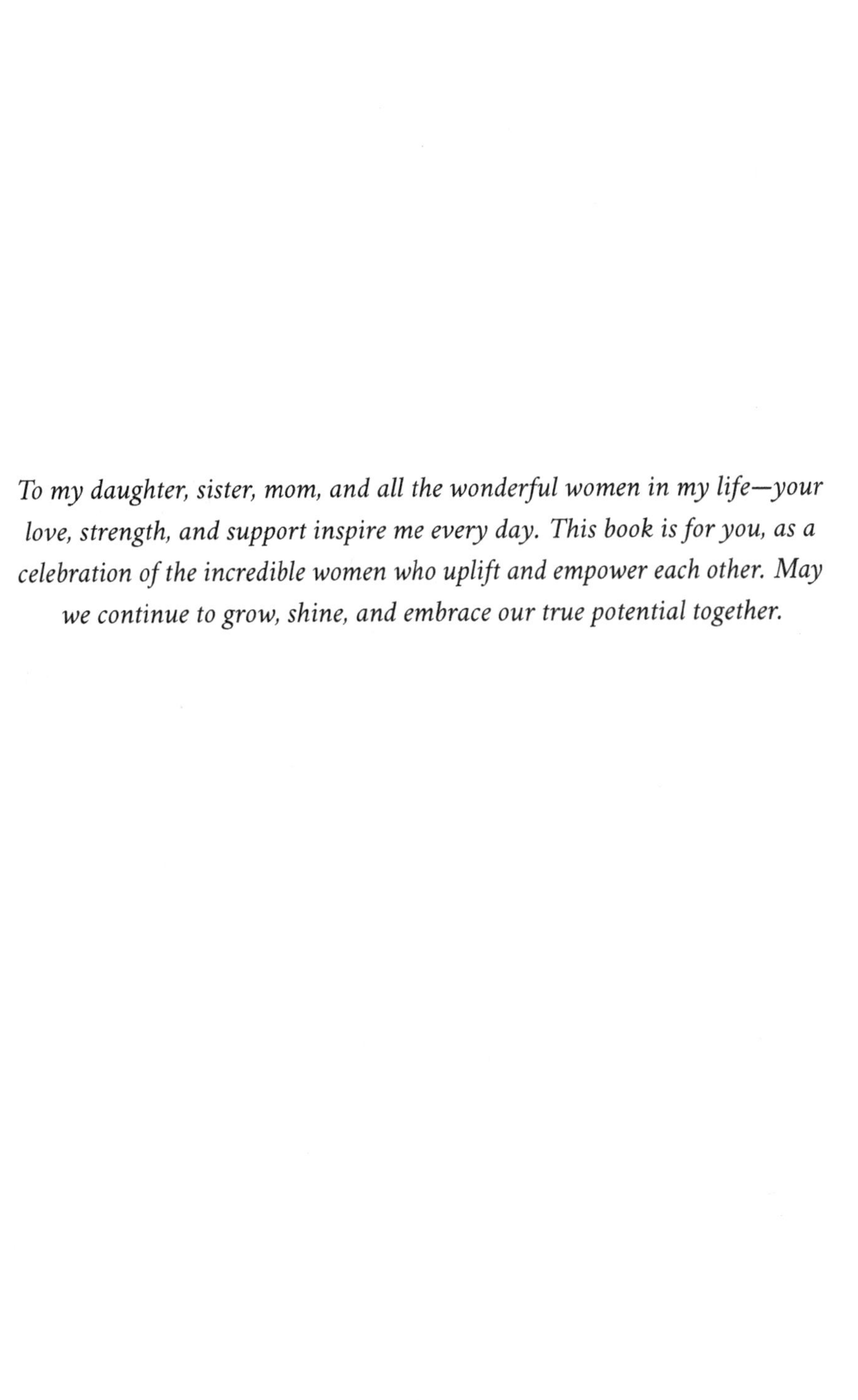

To my daughter, sister, mom, and all the wonderful women in my life—your love, strength, and support inspire me every day. This book is for you, as a celebration of the incredible women who uplift and empower each other. May we continue to grow, shine, and embrace our true potential together.

Contents

1

Introduction

Life as a busy woman often feels like a constant balancing act. Between work, family, and personal responsibilities, finding time for fitness might seem impossible. However, staying fit is not just a luxury, it's a necessity for your physical health, mental well-being, and overall energy levels. Fitness is a powerful tool for managing stress, improving focus, and boosting confidence.

Modern life has introduced us to countless conveniences, but it has also made sedentary behavior more common. Many women find themselves spending hours at a desk or juggling responsibilities, leaving little room for self-care. Yet, fitness doesn't have to be confined to the four walls of a gym. This book dispels the myth that gyms are necessary for fitness. It's a simple, no-frills guide designed to help you stay active, healthy, and energized from the comfort of your home.

In today's world, fitness is often presented as a complex, time-consuming endeavor requiring high-end equipment, trendy classes, or a significant financial investment. However, this book is here to challenge that narrative. It emphasizes simplicity, showing you how to prioritize movement in realistic and practical ways.

Whether your goal is weight loss, increased strength, or improved flexibility, this book will empower you to take charge of your fitness journey—even with a packed schedule. The tools, techniques, and insights shared in this book are tailored for busy women who need practical solutions that work. Each chapter offers actionable advice, true-life examples, and strategies to integrate fitness into your lifestyle seamlessly. Let's dive in and transform the way you think about fitness.

This book is more than just about fitness; it's about reshaping your mindset, taking control of your health, and learning how to incorporate wellness into your busy lifestyle without guilt, stress, or time constraints.

As women, we wear many hats: mother, wife, daughter, friend, professional, and more. It's no wonder that finding time for ourselves can feel impossible. But the truth is, when we prioritize our health, everything else falls into place. You'll have more energy, less stress, improved mental clarity, and confidence that radiates through every aspect of your life. This is not just about weight loss; it's about being the best version of yourself.

In this book, I'll guide you through simple, effective home workouts designed to fit your schedule, no matter how busy you are. You'll learn how to make fitness a daily habit, nourish your body with the right foods, and develop a resilient mindset that supports your journey. So, let's get started.

2

Benefits of Working Out at Home

Home workouts offer a variety of benefits that cater for busy lifestyles:

- **Time-saving:** No need to commute to the gym. The minutes you save can add up to hours each week, allowing you to invest that time in other priorities or simply enjoy a moment of rest. For example, instead of spending 30 minutes driving to and from a gym, you can complete a full workout in that same amount of time.
- **Cost-effective:** Eliminate expensive memberships and equipment. By using your home environment creatively, you can achieve excellent results without spending a fortune. Many online platforms also provide free or low-cost workout videos tailored for home settings.
- **Flexibility:** Exercise whenever it fits your schedule, whether it's early in the morning, during your lunch break, or after the kids are asleep. This flexibility makes it easier to stay consistent, as you aren't bound by gym hours or peak times.

- **Privacy:** Work out in the comfort of your own space without judgment. This is particularly valuable for those who feel self-conscious exercising in front of others or for beginners who prefer to try new routines at their own pace.

Real-life example: Maria, a mother of two, used to struggle with gym commitments. By switching to home workouts, she managed to save over $500 annually on gym fees and discovered she could squeeze in a 20-minute routine while her kids napped. Her new approach not only helped her stay fit but also allowed her to be present at home.

3

What You'll Need For Home Workout

You don't need a fully equipped gym to start. Here's a list of basic essentials and why they're useful:

• **Yoga mat:** Provides stability and comfort during exercises. It's especially helpful for floor-based activities like stretching or core work. A good-quality mat can also prevent slips and injuries.

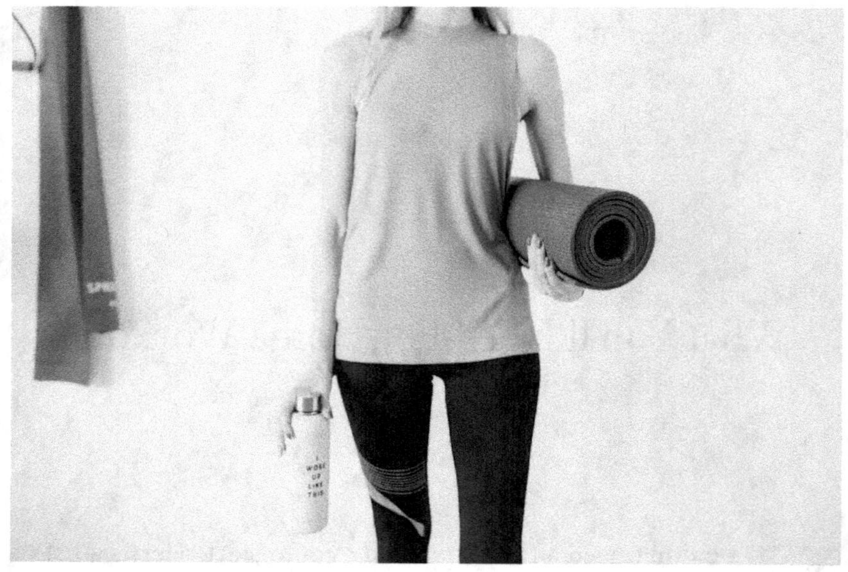

Resistance bands: Versatile tools for strength training. They come in various levels of resistance to match your fitness level. Resistance bands are lightweight and portable, making them ideal for traveling as well.

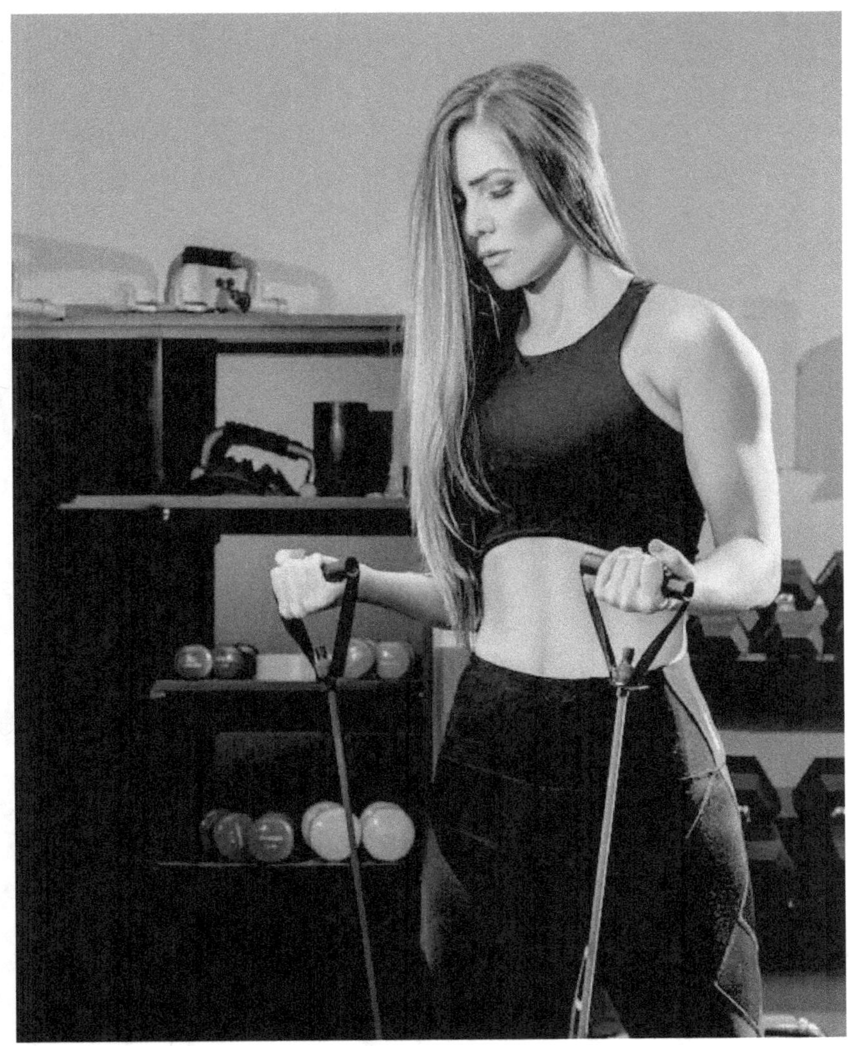

- **Light dumbbells:** Optional but effective for adding resistance to upper body exercises like bicep curls or shoulder presses. For beginners, household items like water bottles or canned goods can serve as substitutes.

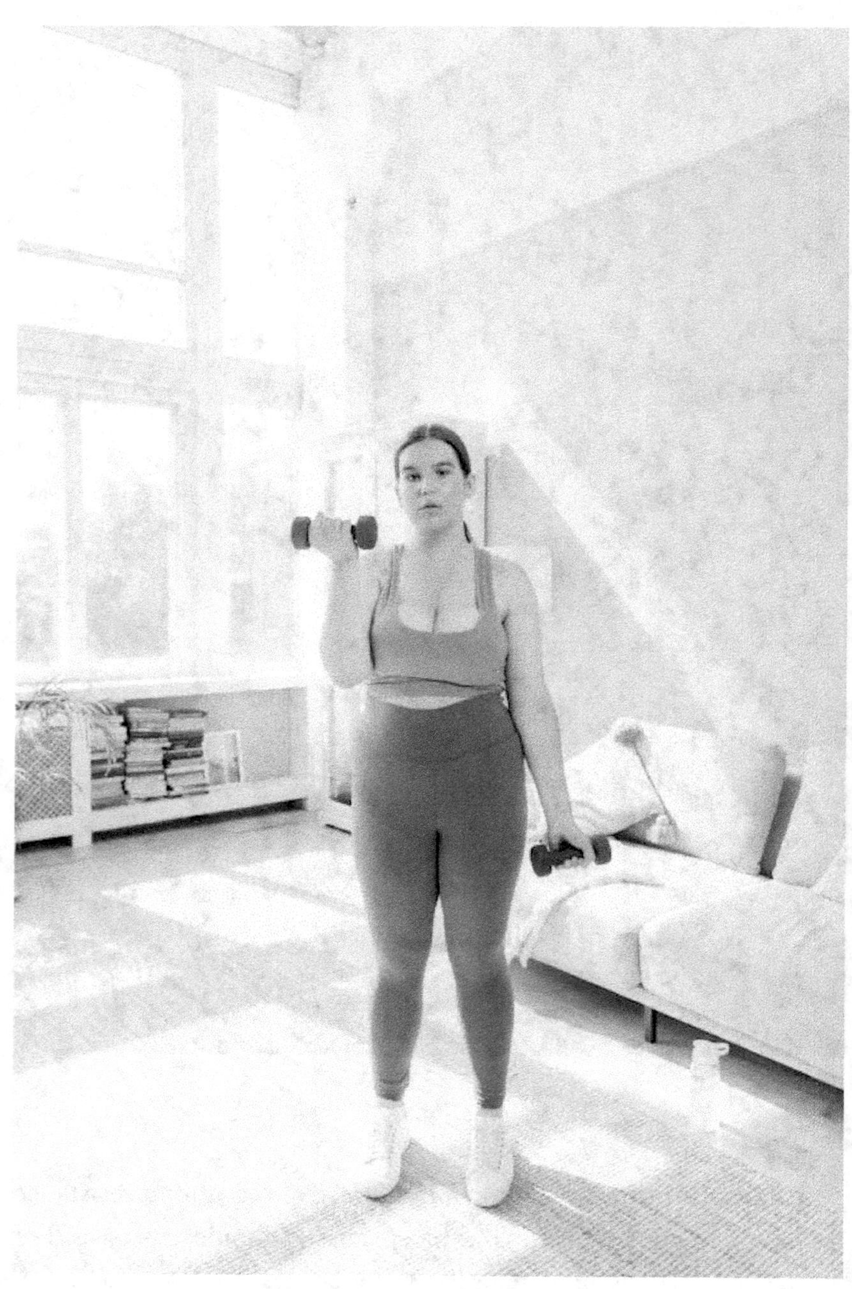

- **Household items:** Use water bottles as weights or a sturdy chair for tricep dips and step-ups. These improvisations can be just as effective as gym equipment and demonstrate that fitness can be resourceful.
- **Comfortable workout clothes and shoes:** Wearing the right gear ensures comfort and reduces the risk of injury. Opt for breathable fabrics and supportive footwear to enhance your workout experience.
- **Walking Pad:** Walking pads are compact, portable treadmills designed for use at home or under a desk. They provide a convenient way to incorporate movement into your day, especially for women who spend long hours sitting.

Incorporating the Walking Pad into Your Day

The walking pad can be easily incorporated into your daily routine without taking up much time. Here's how:

- **While Working:** Set the walking pad up under your desk and walk at a moderate pace (2.5-3.5 mph) for 15-30 minutes at a time while checking emails or working on projects.
- **While Watching TV:** Get in a brisk walk during your favorite show or while listening to a podcast.
- **While Reading or Listening to Audiobooks:** Combine leisure time with exercise for extra steps.

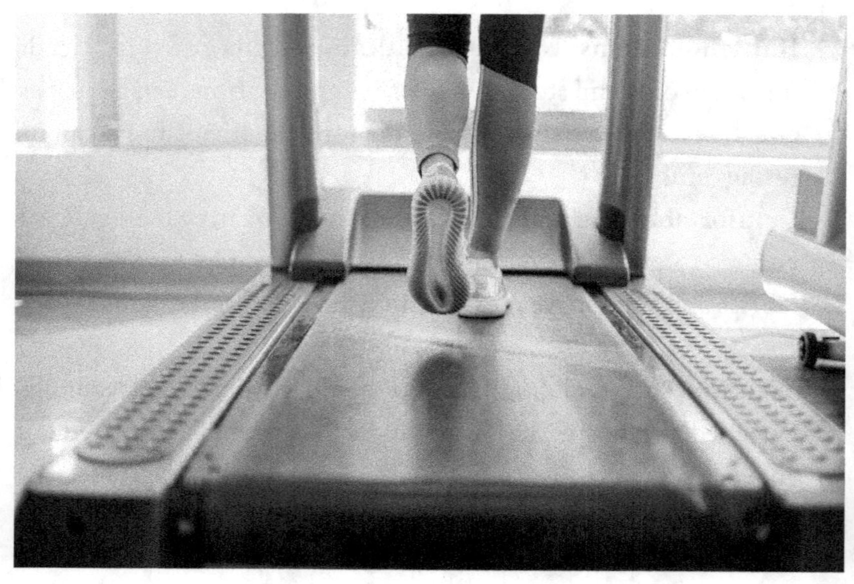

4

Understanding Your Body and Fitness Goals

Understanding your body and setting the right goals is the foundation of a successful fitness journey. Before you dive into any workout routine, it's important to understand where you are right now, where you want to go, and how to measure your progress along the way.

Assessing Your Current Fitness Level

Before starting any new fitness routine, it's essential to assess your current fitness level. This will give you a baseline and help you understand where you're starting from. It will also allow you to track your progress as you go. Here are a few ways to assess your fitness:

1. **Body Measurements**: Take measurements of key areas (waist, hips, chest, arms, and legs). These measurements can be tracked over time to see changes in your body composition.
2. **Fitness Test**: Try basic fitness tests like counting how many squats, push-ups, or burpees you can do in 1 minute. These can help you track endurance and strength progress.

3. **Cardiovascular Endurance**: A simple test is timing yourself while walking or running a mile (or a shorter distance if needed). Repeat this every few weeks to see how much your stamina improves.

4. **Flexibility and Balance**: Test how far you can stretch or how long you can hold balance poses like a tree pose in yoga. Flexibility and balance are just as important as strength in overall fitness.

5

Setting Realistic Goals

Now that you've assessed where you are, it's time to set some goals. Setting clear, achievable goals is crucial for staying motivated and tracking progress. Use the SMART method for setting your goals:

- **Specific:** Be clear about what you want to achieve (e.g., "I want to lose 10 pounds" or "I want to run 2 miles without stopping").
- **Measurable:** Find a way to measure your success (e.g., tracking weight loss or running times).
- **Achievable:** Set goals that are challenging but realistic for your current fitness level.
- **Relevant:** Make sure the goals are meaningful to you (e.g., losing weight for health reasons, or increasing strength for functional fitness).
- **Time-bound:** Set a deadline for achieving your goals (e.g., "I want to lose 10 pounds in the next 3 months").

Short-Term vs. Long-Term Goals

- **Short-term goals**: These are smaller milestones that help you stay on track. For example, committing to a workout routine for 3 weeks or increasing the number of push-ups you can do in a month.
- **Long-term goals**: These are bigger aspirations, like running a 5K, losing 30 pounds, or becoming more flexible. They often take months or years to achieve, but they provide direction for your fitness journey.

Identifying your priorities:

- **Weight loss:** Focus on cardio and high-intensity interval training (HIIT). These exercises are efficient in burning calories and improving heart health.
- **Strength:** Incorporate resistance training to build muscle. Strength training not only tones your body but also improves bone density and metabolic rate.
- **Flexibility:** Include yoga and stretching routines for a balanced approach to improved flexibility and reduces the risk of injuries and to enhance mobility.

Staying consistent is key. Please make sure to set goals that are achievable, such as exercising at least three times a week, and gradually build up. For example, aim to complete a 10-minute workout consistently before increasing the duration. Break your goals into smaller milestones, like completing a week of scheduled workouts or mastering a specific exercise form. Celebrate small wins to maintain motivation, such as being able to do one more push-up or holding a plank for an extra few seconds.

Fitness isn't just about the numbers on the scale. It's about building a strong, resilient body that allows you to live your life fully. Focus on how your body feels rather than how it looks. Can you carry your groceries more easily? Do you have more energy throughout the day? Celebrate those wins, and be patient with the process.

6

The Mindset Shift

Overcoming mental blocks is essential:

- **Combat perfectionism:** Progress, not perfection, matters most. Understand that missing a workout doesn't mean failure—it's an opportunity to start fresh the next day. Embrace the idea that every small effort contributes to long-term success.
  - **Build self-discipline:** Treat workouts as non-negotiable appointments with yourself. Consider them an investment in your health and happiness. Schedule them on your calendar as you would any other important meeting.
  - **Celebrate progress:** Acknowledge even small achievements, like sticking to a routine for a week or trying a new exercise. These moments build confidence and momentum.

Real-life tip: Keep a journal where you log not just your workouts but also how you feel afterward. Tracking your mood and energy levels can be a powerful motivator. For instance, you might notice that your energy levels are consistently higher on days when you exercise, reinforcing the positive habit.

True Life Story: Jessica's Home Workout Breakthrough

Jessica, a 28-year-old teacher, was looking for a workout routine that didn't require a lot of time or equipment. With a small apartment and limited space, she struggled to commit to a gym membership. After discovering bodyweight exercises, Jessica began incorporating them into her daily routine. Push-ups, squats, lunges, and planks became her go-to exercises.

In just six weeks, Jessica noticed increased muscle tone, more energy, and better posture. She was amazed that such effective workouts could be done with nothing more than her own body. Bodyweight training helped Jessica achieve results without any equipment or the need to leave home.

7

Simple and Effective Workouts

1. **Full-Body Engagement**: These exercises work multiple muscle groups simultaneously, increasing calorie burn and muscle development.
2. **Convenient and Accessible**: No need for gym equipment. You can do these exercises anywhere—at home, on vacation, or in the office.
3. **Scalable**: Bodyweight exercises can be made easier depending on your fitness level.

A quick, equipment-free routine to fit into busy mornings:

1. **Bodyweight Squats** – 10-15 repeats (reps). Strengthen your lower body and engage your core.

- **How to do it**: Stand with feet hip-width apart, bend your knees and push your hips back as if you're sitting in a chair. Keep your chest lifted and your knees aligned over your toes. Return to standing.

- **Variations**: Add a jump for a plyometric squat or hold a squat for 30 seconds for a static hold.

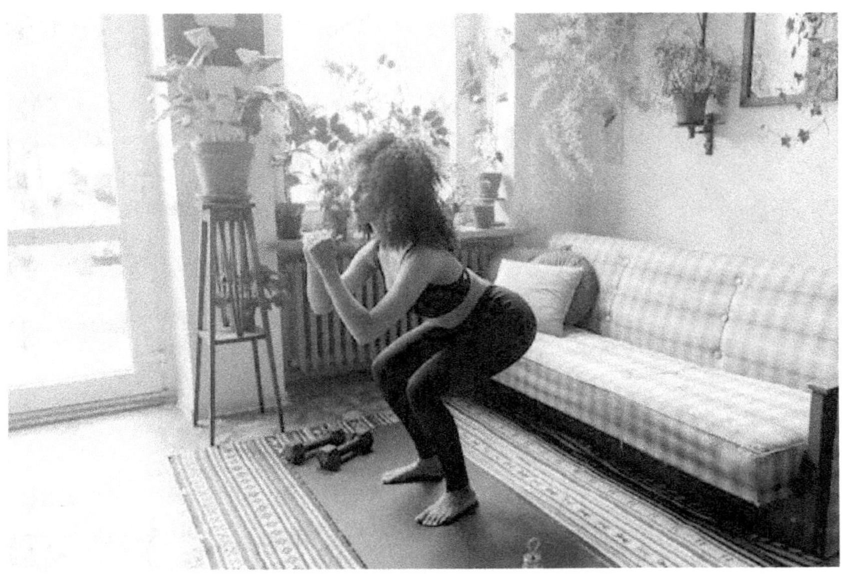

1.
2. **Push-Ups** – 10-15 reps (modify by doing them on your knees). These target your chest, shoulders, and triceps. Ensure proper form by keeping your body in a straight line.

- **How to do it**: Start in a plank position with your hands under your shoulders. Lower your chest toward the floor, then push back up to starting position.
- **Variations**: Start on your knees if you're a beginner, or do incline push-ups using a bench or chair. Progress to full push-ups as you get stronger.

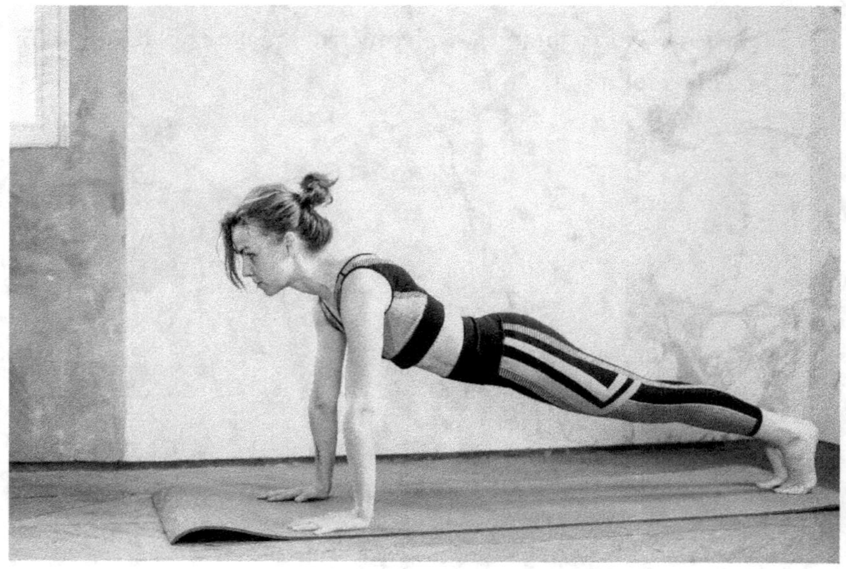

3. Plank – Hold for 30 seconds. Build core stability and strengthen your shoulders. If 30 seconds is challenging, start with 10 seconds and gradually increase.

- **How to do it**: Start in a forearm plank position, keeping your body straight and engaging your core. Hold for as long as possible.

Variations: Add leg lifts or arm reaches to increase the challenge.

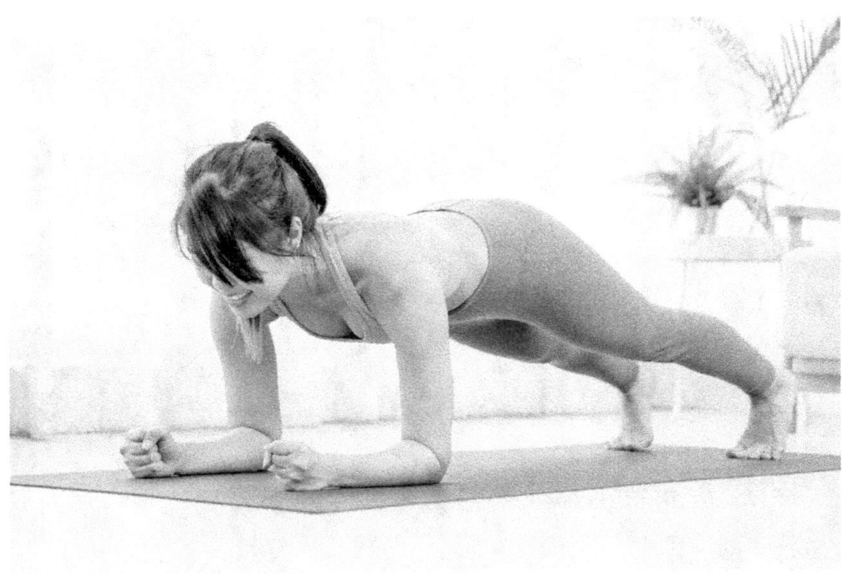

•

4. Jumping Jacks – 20 reps. Get your heart rate up and warm up your entire body. This exercise is a great way to transition into more vigorous activity.

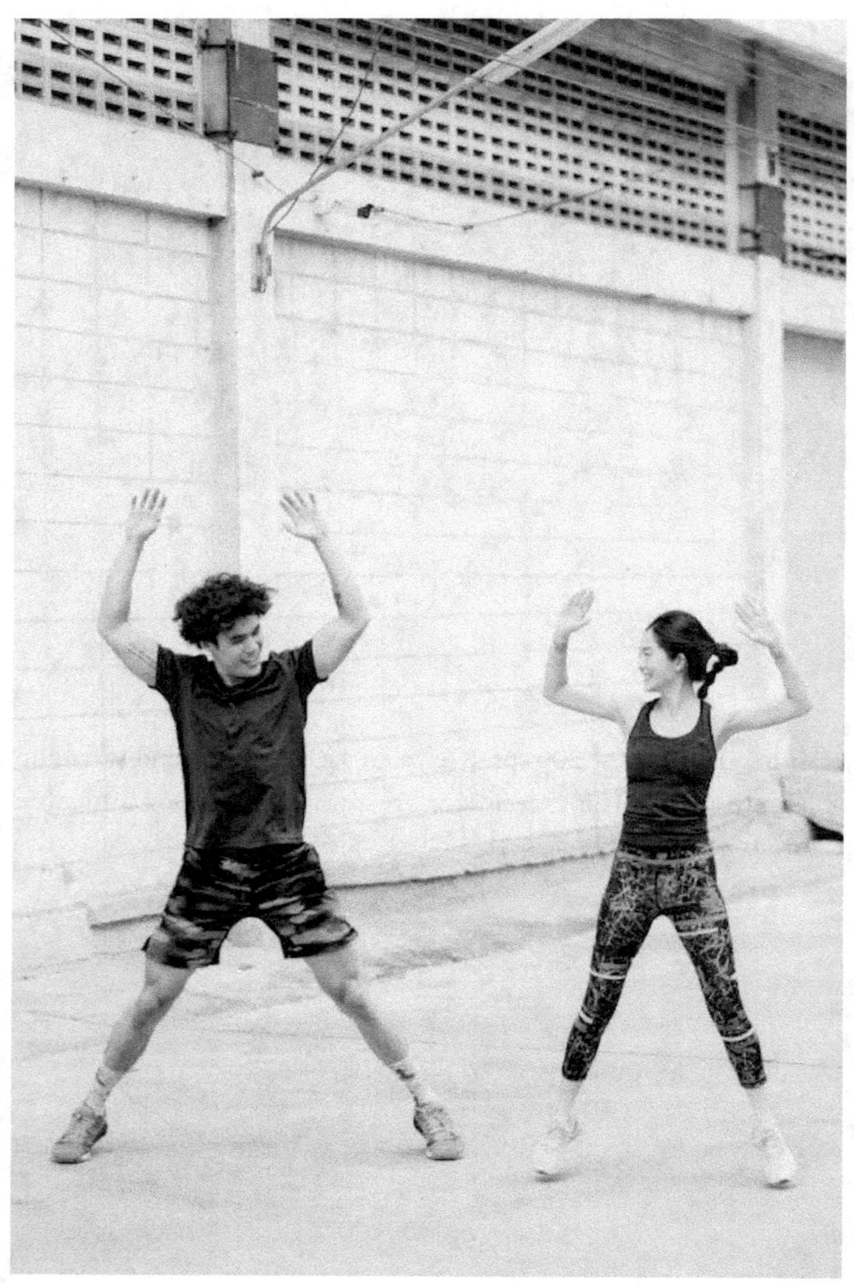

5. Glute Bridges

- **How to do it**: Lie on your back with your knees bent and feet flat on the floor. Lift your hips up towards the ceiling, squeezing your glutes, and slowly lower back down.
- **Variations**: Try single-leg glute bridges or hold at the top for added intensity.

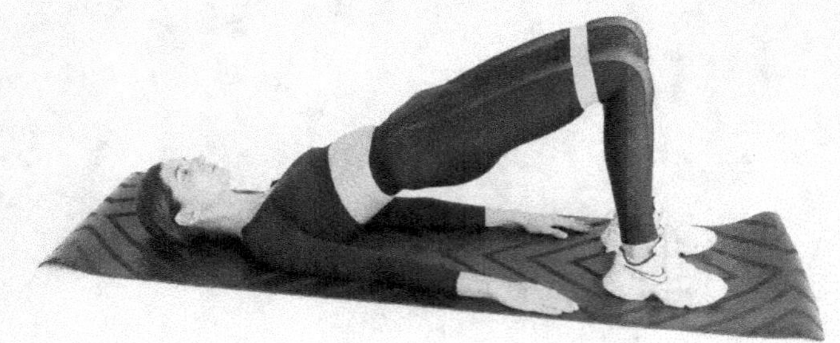

6. Lunges

- **How to do it**: Take a large step forward with one leg, lowering your body until both knees are at 90 degrees. Push back to standing, then repeat on the other side.
- **Variations**: Try reverse lunges or jump lunges for more intensity.

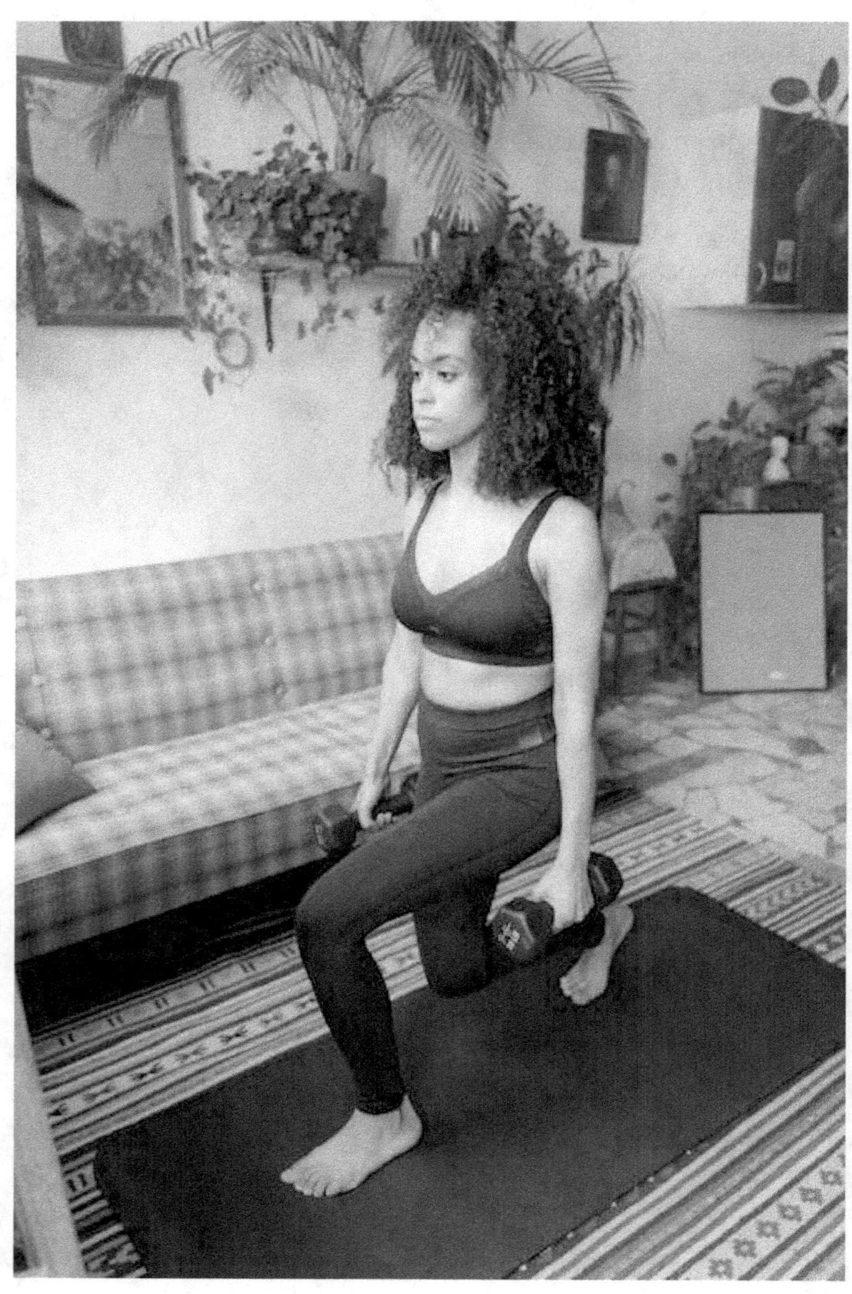

Repeat the circuit twice for an effective workout in just 15 minutes. Customize the routine by increasing reps or adding a third round as you progress.

Targeted Workouts

If you prefer focusing on specific areas, these routines will help:

- **Upper Body:**
- Push-ups (standard or modified) – Strengthen chest and arms.
- Tricep dips using a sturdy chair – Target the back of your arms.
- Shoulder taps in a plank position – Build stability and core strength.
- **Lower Body:**
- Squats – Strengthen thighs and glutes.
- Lunges – Improve balance and tone your legs.
- Glute bridges – Strengthen the lower back and glutes.
- **Core Strength:**
- Planks – Engage the entire core.
- Bicycle crunches – Target obliques.
- Leg raises – Strengthen lower abs.

8

Cardio Workouts That Work for Busy Women

Cardiovascular exercise is essential for heart health, weight management, and overall well-being. But for busy women, finding time for cardio can be a challenge. The good news is, you don't need a lot of time or a gym membership to get a solid cardio workout.

Effective Cardio Options for Busy Women

Cardio doesn't necessarily require a treadmill or elliptical. Try these fun, high-energy alternatives:

- **HIIT:** These workouts alternate between intense activity and rest. Alternate 30 seconds of high-intensity exercises like burpees with 30 seconds of rest. Repeat for 10-15 minutes. **(High-Intensity Interval Training)**: This is a form of cardio that alternates between short bursts of intense exercise and short periods of rest. HIIT can be done in as little as 20 minutes but is highly effective for fat loss and cardiovascular health.

- Example HIIT workout: 30 seconds of jumping jacks, 30 seconds of rest, 30 seconds of burpees, 30 seconds of rest. Repeat for 20 minutes.
- **Dancing:** Put on your favorite music and dance and dance around the house for a full-body cardio session. It's a fun way to get your heart pumping and burn calories.
- **Shadowboxing:** Punch and move as if sparring an imaginary opponent.
- **Walking or Jogging**: Walking is a low-impact but effective cardio workout, it is also one of the simplest ways to get cardio. You can walk or jog on a treadmill, outside in the park, or around your neighborhood. It has a very low-impact and can be done at your own pace. Aim for 30 minutes per day, or break it into smaller sessions.
- **Walking Tip**: Aim for 10,000 steps a day or more. Use a pedometer or a fitness app to track your steps.
- **Jump Rope**: Jumping rope is an excellent cardio workout that requires minimal space and equipment. A few minutes of jumping rope can burn as many calories as running. This fun and affordable cardio workout can burn hundreds of calories in just 15 minutes.
- **Cycling**: Whether it's on a stationary bike or out on the road, cycling is a great low-impact cardio workout.

The Benefits of Cardio

1. **Burns Calories**: Cardio is one of the best ways to burn calories and support weight loss.
2. **Boosts Mood**: Cardiovascular exercise triggers the release of endorphins, which can reduce stress and improve your mood.
3. **Increases Endurance**: Regular cardio increases your stamina,

allowing you to do everyday tasks with more energy.

4. **Improves Heart Health**: Strengthens the heart and improves circulation, reducing the risk of heart disease.
5. **Boosts Lung Capacity**: Enhances respiratory efficiency and oxygen intake.
6. **Aids in Weight Management**: Burns calories and supports healthy weight loss or maintenance.
7. **Improves Sleep**: Promotes better sleep quality and regulates sleep cycles.
8. **Enhances Metabolism**: Encourages efficient calorie burning and fat metabolism.

Time-Efficient Cardio Routines

If you're pressed for time, try this 15-minute HIIT workout:

- 1 minute of high knees
- 1 minute of mountain climbers
- 1 minute of jumping jacks
- 1 minute of burpees
- Repeat 3 times with 30 seconds of rest in between each round.

This short routine burns a lot of calories and gets your heart rate up quickly.

True Life Story: Linda's Quick Cardio Solution

Linda, a 45-year-old lawyer, spent long hours at her desk and often felt drained by the end of the day. She knew that she needed to include cardio in her routine, but she couldn't find the time for long workouts. After trying a few quick HIIT (High-Intensity Interval

Training) routines, she was hooked. In just 20 minutes, she was able to elevate her heart rate and burn calories. As her fitness level increased, she began to feel more energized and less stressed.

Linda's success story proves that even a short, intense burst of cardio can make a significant difference.

9

Basic Flexibility and Stretching Exercises

Incorporating Flexibility and Balance

Many women focus on strength and cardio, but flexibility and recovery are equally important. Stretching and yoga are key for reducing muscle tension, improving range of motion, and preventing injury.

Incorporate stretching and flexibility exercises into your daily routine to support a healthier and more active lifestyle is very important, it helps enhance your mobility, making everyday movements easier and more comfortable to prepared you for your daily tasks .

Regular stretching also alleviates stress, both physical and mental, promoting relaxation and overall well-being, it helps prevent back pain and enhances your stability leaving you feeling more energized and refreshed throughout the day.

Start with just a few minutes each morning or evening—it's a simple, effective way to care for your body and mind!

Why Stretching/Flexibility Matters

1. **Prepares the Body**: Warms up muscles and increases blood flow.
2. **Prevents Injury**: Stretching before and after workouts helps improve flexibility and reduce the risk of injury, Stretching helps keep muscles and joints flexible, reducing the risk of strains and sprains.
3. **Promotes Relaxation**: Gentle stretches can lower stress and ease muscle tightness.
4. **Improves Posture**: Stretching can alleviate tight muscles and improve spinal alignment. Flexibility exercises also help keep your spine aligned and prevent discomfort.
5. **Boosts Circulation**: Promotes oxygen delivery to muscles, improving efficiency.
6. **Mental Focus**: Helps shift your mindset to the upcoming activity, enhancing concentration.
7. **Promotes Recovery**: Reduces muscle tension and soreness by encouraging relaxation and circulation.
8. **Aids in Cooling Down**: Helps bring heart rate and breathing back to normal after exercise.

Stretching and Relaxation Techniques

- **Dynamic Stretching**: Warm up your muscles before a workout with dynamic movements like arm circles or leg swings.
- **Post-Workout Stretching**: Cool down with static stretches to release tension in your muscles.
- **Relaxation Practices**: Incorporate yoga, deep breathing, or meditation to enhance recovery.
- *Actionable Tip*: Dedicate 10 minutes before bedtime to a stretching routine focused on tight areas like your shoulders and lower back.

True Life Story: Nicole's Yoga Journey

Nicole, a 32-year-old mother of three, experienced chronic back pain from sitting at a desk all day. After a visit to her chiropractor, she was advised to add flexibility training to her routine. Nicole began practicing yoga, focusing on gentle stretches to alleviate muscle tension. Over time, she noticed a decrease in her back pain and a marked improvement in her overall flexibility.

Nicole's story highlights the importance of incorporating recovery and flexibility into your routine, especially for women who spend long hours sitting.

Basic Flexibility and Stretching Exercises

1. **Cat-Cow Stretch**: On your hands and knees, arch your back (cat), then dip it toward the floor while lifting your head (cow). Repeat 10 times.
2. **Downward Dog**: Start in a plank position and push your hips up toward the ceiling, forming an inverted V. Hold for 30 seconds.
3. **Child's Pose**: Sit on your knees, stretch your arms forward, and lower your chest toward the ground. Hold for 30 seconds.
4. **Forward Fold**: Stand with feet hip-width apart, fold forward from the hips, and reach for your toes. Hold for 30 seconds.
5. **Basic Yoga Poses:** Yoga and stretching can lower stress levels and calm the mind as well, e.g. warrior pose improves flexibility and focus. Yoga is not only great for flexibility but also for mental clarity. Here's a simple 15-minute routine you can do after your workout or in the evening to unwind.

It is very important to always balance your daily routine with stretches and low-impact exercises.

Simple Yoga Routine for Flexibility

- Cat-Cow Stretch (1 minute)

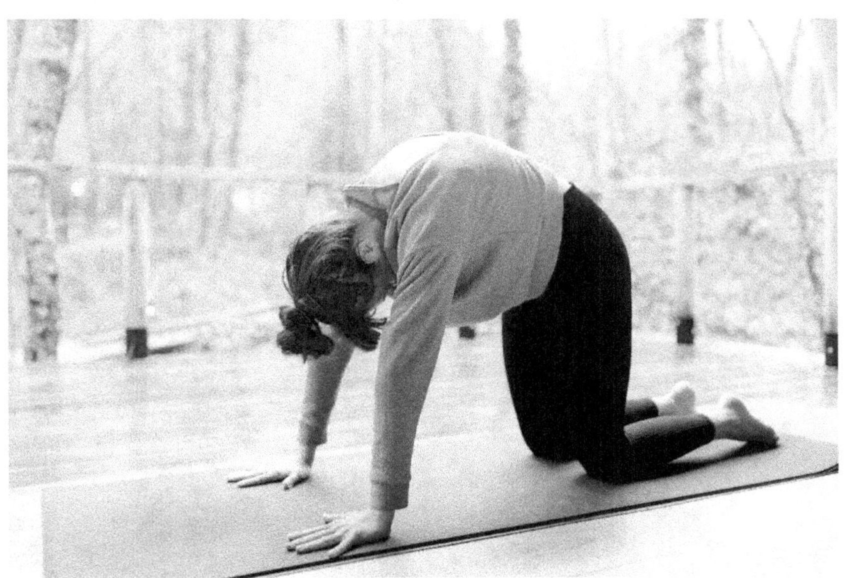

- Downward Dog (1 minute)

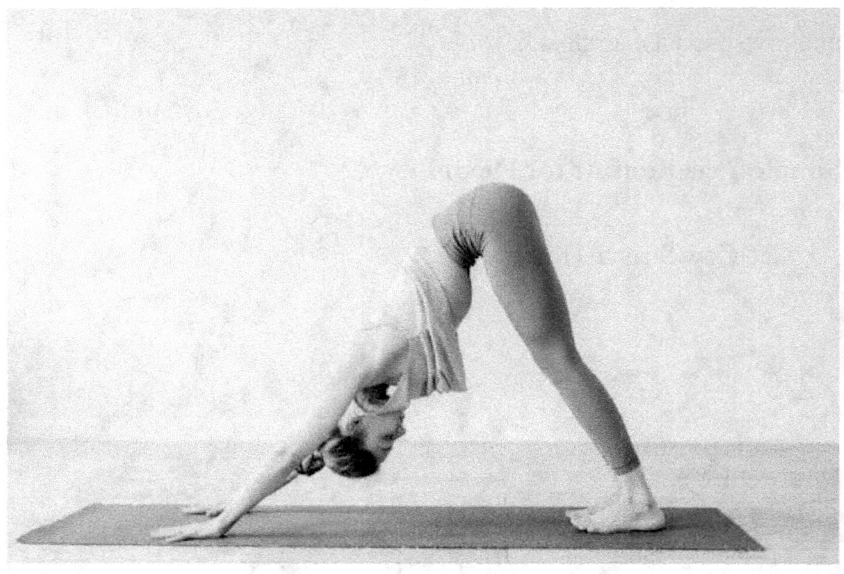

• Forward Fold (1 minute)

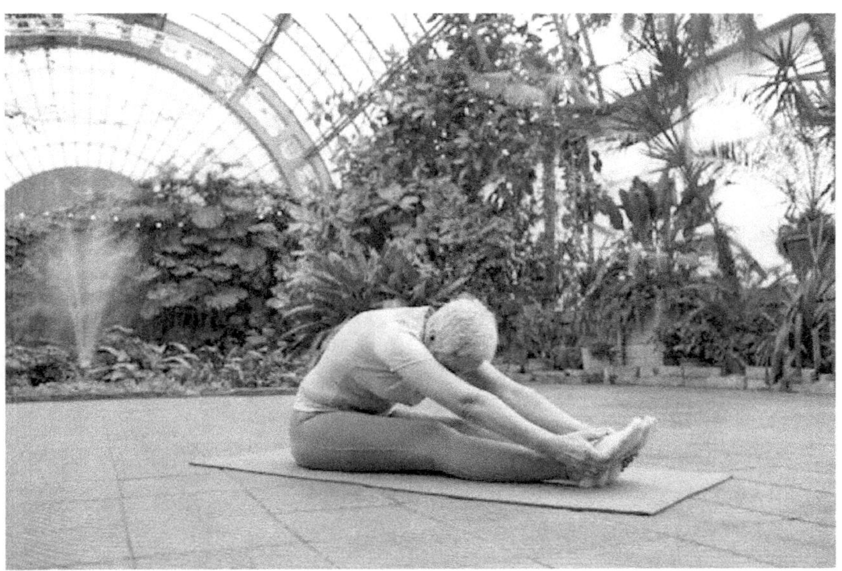

- Child's Pose (1 minute)

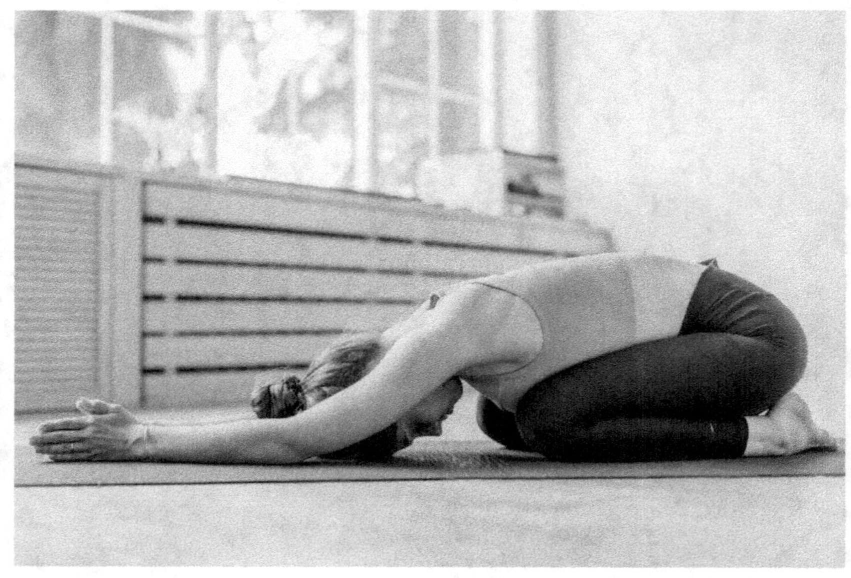

- Seated Forward Bend (2 minutes)

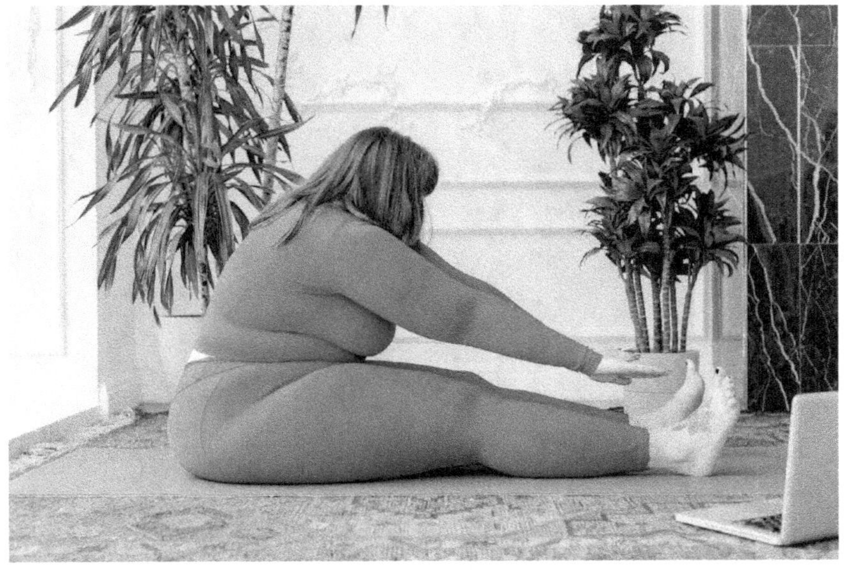

- Supine Twist (2 minutes)

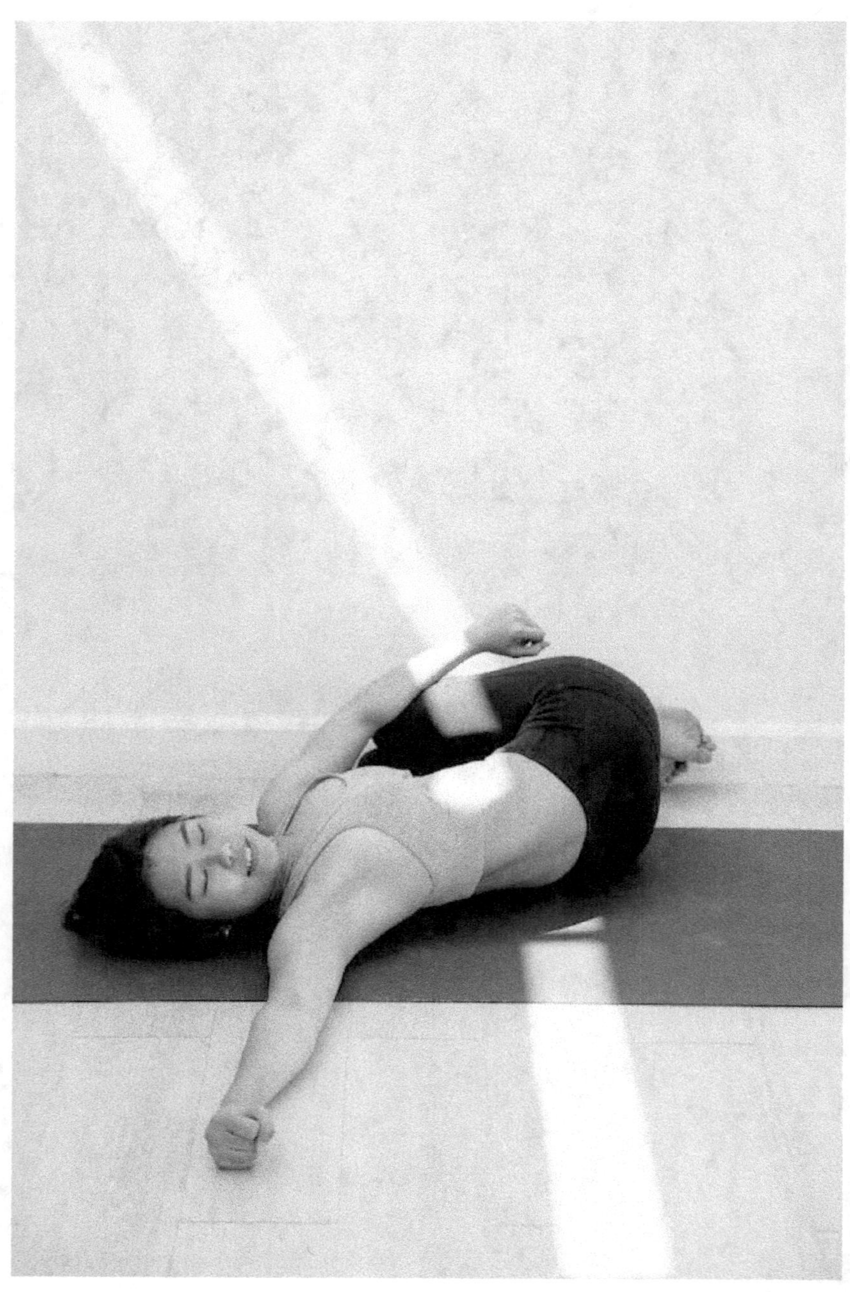

- **Stretching Routines:** Dedicate 5-10 minutes after a workout to stretch major muscle groups.

41

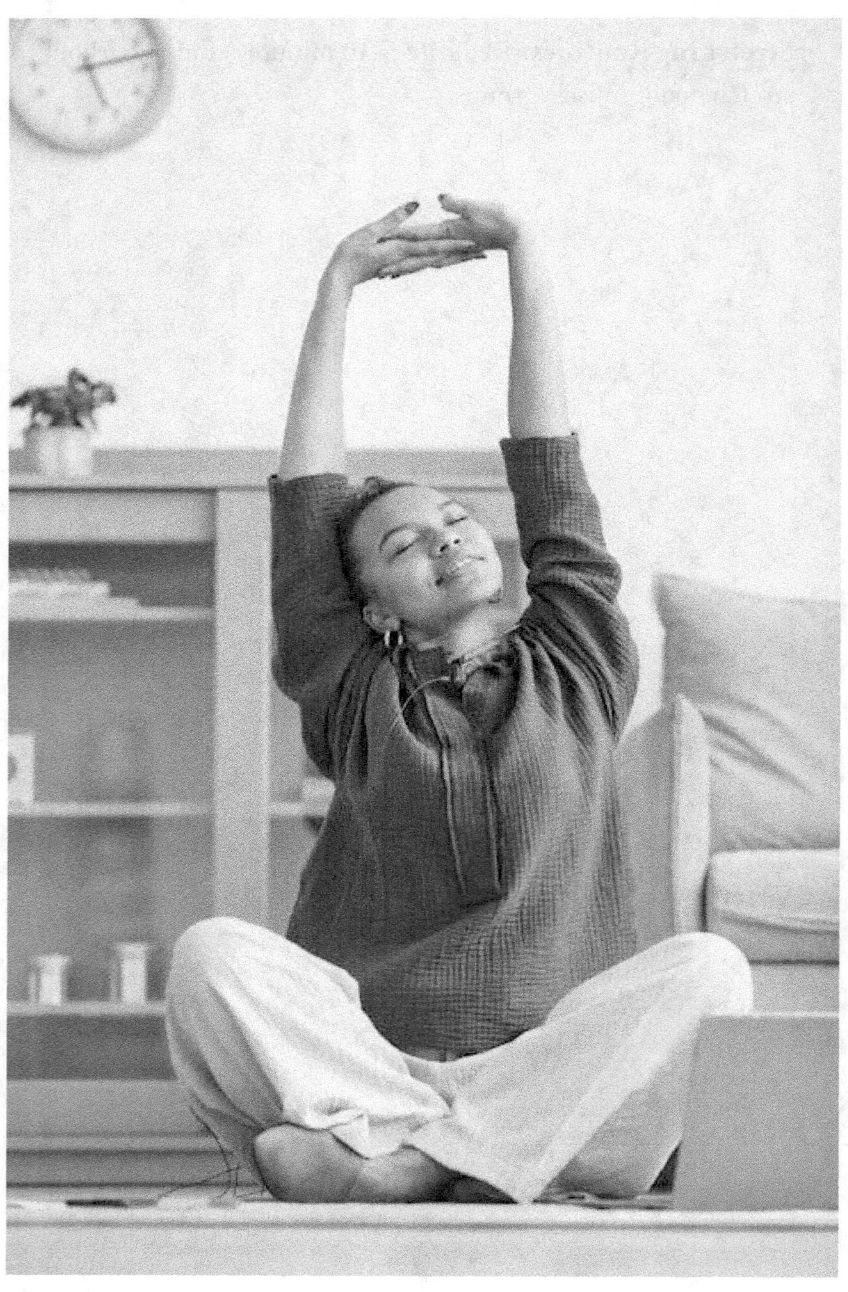

- **Pilates Moves:** Try leg circles or the hundred for core and flexibility.

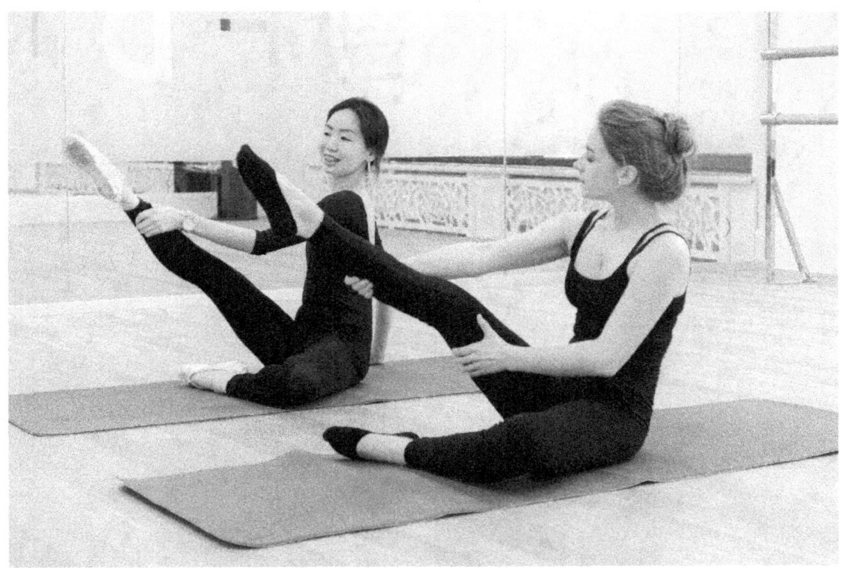

Involving Family and Pets-Fitness can also be a shared experience:

- **Involving Kids:** Turn playtime into workout time by doing exercises together, like races or jumping jacks.

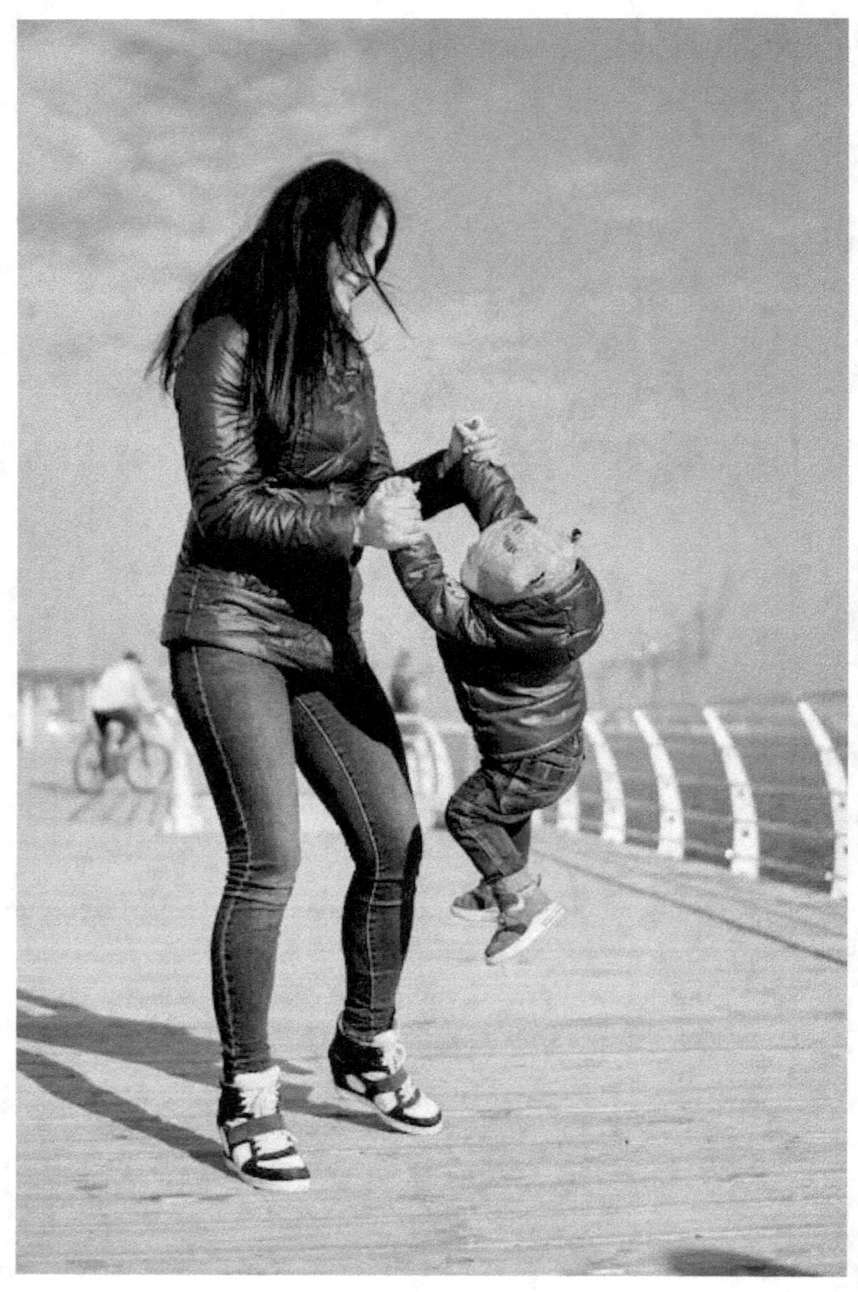

- **Including Pets**: Go for a jog or long walk with your dog to combine exercise with quality time.

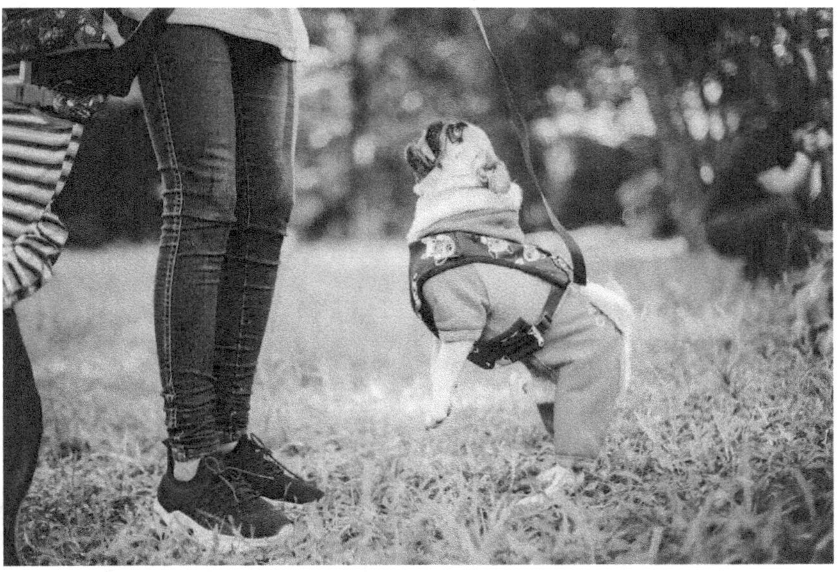

This collaborative approach makes fitness more enjoyable and helps you stay accountable.

10

Creating a Workout Routine That Fits Your Busy Life

Creating a workout routine that fits seamlessly into your busy schedule is key to success. Life is unpredictable, and we're often juggling multiple roles. The key is to design a workout routine that's flexible, efficient, and realistic.

Staying consistent with a fitness routine can be challenging, especially when juggling multiple responsibilities. But consistency is key to seeing progress and making fitness a sustainable part of your lifestyle. This chapter will explore strategies to help you stay on track, measure progress effectively, and maintain motivation.

Creating a sustainable workout routine is key to long-term success. Start by evaluating your daily schedule and identifying windows of opportunity for exercise. Even as little as 15 minutes a day can yield significant benefits over time.

Here are some tips:

- **Identify Your Peak Energy Times**: Determine whether you have more energy in the morning, afternoon, or evening. Schedule your workouts accordingly to maximize efficiency.

- *True-Life Example*: Sarah, a busy mom and marketing professional, found that exercising early in the morning before her kids woke up helped her stay consistent. By waking up 30 minutes earlier, she could complete a 15-minute workout and start her day feeling accomplished.
- **Break It Down**: Don't aim for hour-long sessions if you don't have the time. Short, focused workouts can be just as effective.
- *Actionable Tip*: Try 10-minute intervals of movement throughout the day—a quick walk, squats while brushing your teeth, or desk stretches.
- **Create a Schedule**: Use a planner or app to block out workout times. Treat these appointments as non-negotiable.

See other options below:

- **Morning Workouts:** Exercising early can energize you for the rest of the day. Set your alarm 20 minutes earlier and prepare your workout clothes the night before to streamline the process.
- **Lunchtime Sessions:** Use part of your lunch break to squeeze in a quick workout. A brisk walk or a short HIIT session can revitalize your afternoon.
- **Evening Wind-Downs:** If mornings are too hectic, end your day with yoga or stretching exercises to relax and DE-stress.

Experiment with different times to discover what works best for you. The key is to remain flexible and adapt your routine as needed.

Tracking Progress:

Measuring your progress keeps you motivated and focused. However, it's important not to fixate solely on the scale.

Measuring your progress doesn't have to revolve around the scale. Here are practical ways to track improvement:

- **Performance Metrics**: Note how many push-ups, squats, or planks you can do at the beginning and check your progress weekly.
- *True-Life Example*: Maria, a freelance designer, celebrated her first 30-second plank and increased to a minute after three weeks. Seeing her strength improve motivated her to keep going.
- **Visual Changes**: Take progress photos monthly to observe subtle changes in your body.
- **Mood and Energy Levels**: Pay attention to how regular exercise improves your mental clarity and energy throughout the day.

See more options below:

Designing a Weekly Workout Plan is not a bad idea.

The key to success they say is consistency. But consistency doesn't mean working out every day for hours. Instead, it's about creating a weekly plan that works for your life. Here's a simple weekly template:

- **Monday**: Strength training (lower body) + flexibility
- **Tuesday**: Cardio (HIIT or moderate-intensity) + recovery (light stretching or yoga)
- **Wednesday**: Strength training (upper body) + core work
- **Thursday**: Cardio (walking, cycling, or swimming) + flexibility
- **Friday**: Total body strength workout + recovery
- **Saturday**: Active rest (walking, or dancing)
- **Sunday**: Rest day or light stretching

Time-Saving Tips for Busy Women

- **Use Short, Intense Workouts**: If you're short on time, try high-intensity interval training (HIIT). HIIT involves short bursts of intense exercise followed by brief rest periods. It's proven to burn fat and improve cardiovascular fitness in less time than traditional workouts.
- **Micro Workouts**: If you can't commit to a full workout session, break it up. Try 5-10 minutes of exercise multiple times throughout the day (e.g., 10-minute workout in the morning, 10 minutes after lunch, and 10 minutes before dinner).
- **Workouts on the Go**: Utilize spare moments during your day to sneak in some fitness. Do squats while waiting for your coffee, lunges during TV commercials, or calf raises while brushing your teeth.

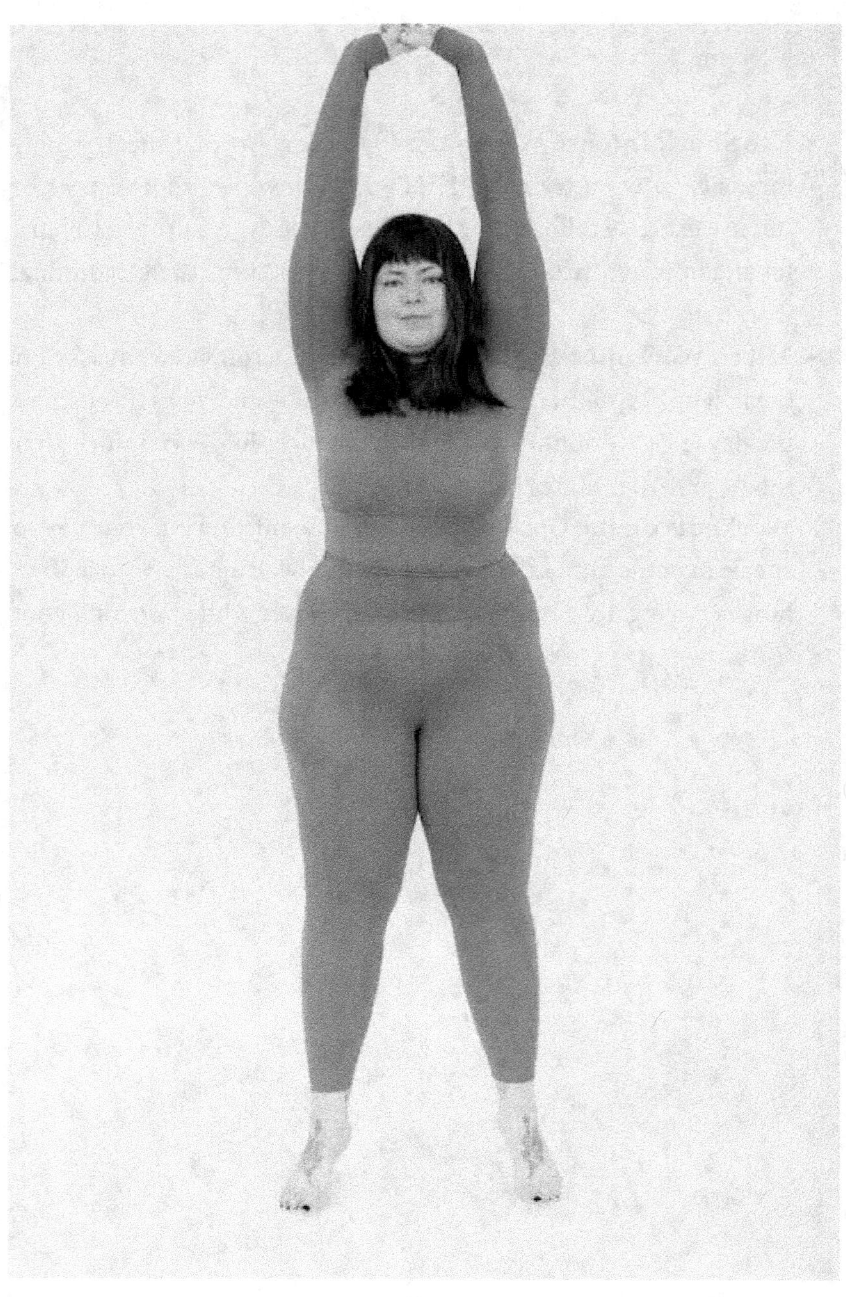

Calf Raises

Creating Flexibility in Your Routine

Sometimes, life gets in the way. Kids get sick, work emergencies arise, or your energy level is low. This is where flexibility comes in.

- **Plan for "bad days"**: It's okay to miss a workout. Instead of feeling discouraged, move on and adjust. Maybe you need a gentler day of yoga instead of an intense cardio session. Allow yourself grace.
- **Alternate workouts**: If you miss a workout, simply swap it for another day. The most important thing is to keep going and not let a missed day derail your progress.

Staying Motivated.

Motivation can wane, but these strategies can help you reignite your drive:

- **Find Your "Why"**: Reflect on the deeper reasons for staying active, such as being a role model for your kids or improving your health.
- **Set Milestones and Rewards**: Celebrate small victories, like completing a week of workouts, by treating yourself to something enjoyable (e.g., a new book or a relaxing bath).
- **Join Support Groups**: Connect with online fitness communities or start a group with friends, church members, classmates and any group you belong to, to share your progress and stay accountable.
- *True-Life Example*: When Lisa joined an online group for women balancing careers and fitness, she found encouragement and new ideas for workouts that fit her schedule.

11

Making Fitness a Lifestyle

Fitness is more than just a goal—it's a way of life. When you make fitness a lifestyle, it becomes an integral part of your daily routine, not just something you do occasionally or as a short-term challenge. It's about creating habits that support your physical and mental well-being, embracing movement in ways you enjoy, and building a sustainable relationship with exercise and healthy living.

The beauty of making fitness a lifestyle is that it adapts to your unique needs and preferences. Whether it's a brisk morning walk, a yoga session to unwind, or a strength workout to feel empowered, the key is consistency and balance. This approach not only enhances your physical health but also boosts your energy, sharpens your focus, and uplifts your mood, empowering you to lead a more vibrant and fulfilling life.

Ready to embrace fitness as a lifestyle? Let's explore how small, consistent steps can lead to long-lasting change!

The ultimate goal is to integrate movement into your daily life effortlessly. Fitness shouldn't feel like a chore—it should become a natural part of your routine.

Incorporating Movement into Daily Life

Small changes can make a big difference:

- **Walk More**: Park farther away, take the stairs, or set a reminder to move every hour.
- *True-Life Example*: Rajni, a busy accountant, used her lunch breaks for brisk walks and noticed significant improvements in her energy levels.
- **Active Chores**: Turn cleaning, gardening, or organizing into calorie-burning activities.

Turning Short Breaks into Mini Fitness Sessions

Use breaks as opportunities to stay active:

- **Desk Exercises**: Try seated leg lifts, shoulder rolls, or stretches.
- **5-Minute Boosts**: Do a quick set of squats, lunges, or jumping jacks during commercial breaks or between tasks.
- *Actionable Tip*: Keep resistance bands near your workspace for quick strength-building exercises.

Building a Supportive Environment

Create a space and community that fosters a fitness-friendly lifestyle:

- **Dedicated Workout Area**: Set up a corner with your mat, weights, or bands to encourage daily exercise.
- **Family Involvement**: Get your kids or partner involved in fun activities like dancing, hiking, or outdoor games.
- *True-Life Example*: Elena started weekend dance-offs with her kids,

turning family time into a calorie-burning activity.

12

Nutrition and Fitness

While exercise is vital, nutrition plays an equally important role in achieving fitness goals. Eating the right foods is crucial for supporting your fitness routine and maintaining a healthy lifestyle. As a busy woman, it can be easy to fall into the trap of grabbing unhealthy snacks or skipping meals. The key is to make nutrition simple, balanced, and sustainable.

True Life Story: Kate's Meal Prep Success story

Kate, a 37-year-old project manager, often found herself grabbing unhealthy snacks between meetings. She knew that to maintain energy throughout the day, she needed to improve her nutrition. Kate started meal prepping on Sundays, cooking batches of healthy meals for the week. With meals ready to go, she stopped relying on takeout and snacks, feeling more energized and focused at work.

Kate's success shows how small changes in meal prep can make a big difference in your daily nutrition.

Essential Nutrients for Women

1. **Protein**: Helps with muscle repair and growth. Good sources include chicken, fish, tofu, beans, and eggs.
2. **Healthy Fats**: Important for hormone regulation and overall health. Avocados, nuts, seeds, and olive oil are great sources.
3. **Carbohydrates**: Fuel for your workouts. Choose whole grains, fruits, and vegetables over refined sugars and processed foods.
4. **Fiber**: Aids in digestion and keeps you full longer. Include fiber-rich foods like vegetables, fruits, and whole grains.

Quick, Healthy Meal Ideas for Busy Women

1. **Breakfast**: Greek yogurt with fruit and granola or a smoothie with protein powder, spinach, and almond milk.
2. **Lunch**: Salad with lean protein (chicken, tuna, or chickpeas), avocado, and a light vinaigrette dressing.
3. **Dinner**: Grilled salmon with roasted vegetables and quinoa.
4. **Snacks**: Apple slices with almond butter, mixed nuts, or a protein bar.

Here are some easy-to-implement tips:

- **Meal Prepping for Busy Women**: If you don't have time to cook every day, meal prep is a game-changer. Dedicate an hour on the weekend prepping your meals or snacks for the week. Cook a large batch of chicken, quinoa, or vegetables and portion them into containers for easy grab-and-go meals.
- *True-Life Example*: Jenna, a teacher, saved time and stayed on track by preparing overnight oats and portioning fruits and veggies for snacks.
- **Balanced Eating**: Focus on meals rich in lean protein, whole grains,

healthy fats, and vegetables. Avoid processed foods as much as possible.

- **Quick Recipes for Busy Days**: Try simple meals like grilled chicken salads, veggie stir-fry, or smoothies packed with spinach, fruits, and Greek yogurt.

7-Day Meal Plan for Busy Women

Day 1:

- **Breakfast**: Smoothie with protein powder, spinach, and almond milk.
- **Lunch**: Grilled chicken salad with avocado.
- **Dinner**: Salmon with roasted sweet potatoes.
- **Snack**: Apples

Day 2:

- **Breakfast**: Greek yogurt with granola.
- **Lunch**: Turkey and avocado wrap.
- **Dinner**: Stir-fry with tofu and vegetables.
- **Snack**: Peanut

Day 3:

- **Breakfast**: Overnight oats with chia seeds, almond butter, and banana slices
- **Lunch**: Grilled chicken breast with quinoa and roasted veggies (broccoli, sweet potato, and bell peppers)
- **Dinner**: Baked salmon with steamed asparagus and brown rice

- **Snack**: Hummus and carrot sticks

Day 4:

- **Breakfast**: Scrambled eggs with spinach and avocado
- **Lunch**: Turkey and spinach wrap with a side of mixed fruit
- **Dinner**: Veggie stir-fry with tofu and brown rice
- **Snack**: Greek yogurt with berries and honey

Day 5:

- **Breakfast**: Green smoothie with spinach, banana, protein powder, and almond milk
- **Lunch**: Quinoa salad with chickpeas, cucumbers, tomatoes, and feta cheese
- **Dinner**: Grilled shrimp with zucchini noodles and a lemon-tahini dressing
- **Snack**: A handful of almonds

Day 6 and 7: You may spoil yourself a little

Bonus Section: Healthy Recipes for Busy Women:
Breakfast Recipes:

1. **Avocado Toast with Poached Eggs**Ingredients: Whole-grain bread, 1 ripe avocado, 2 eggs, salt, and pepper.Instructions: Toast the bread, smash the avocado onto the toast, top with a poached egg, and season with salt and pepper.
2. **Spinach and Mushroom Scramble**Ingredients: 2 eggs, 1 cup spinach, ½ cup mushrooms, olive oil, salt, and pepper.Instructions: Sauté mushrooms in olive oil, add spinach, and cook until wilted.

Scramble in eggs and cook until set. Season to taste.

Lunch Recipes:

1. **Grilled Chicken Salad**Ingredients: 2 chicken breasts, mixed greens, cucumber, tomatoes, olive oil, lemon juice.Instructions: Grill chicken until cooked through. Toss with salad ingredients and drizzle with olive oil and lemon juice.
2. **Quinoa and Chickpea Bowl**Ingredients: 1 cup cooked quinoa, ½ cup cooked chickpeas, cucumber, red onion, olive oil, lemon juice.Instructions: Mix quinoa, chickpeas, and veggies. Drizzle with olive oil and lemon juice. Serve chilled.

Dinner Recipes:

1. **Baked Salmon with Veggies**Ingredients: 2 salmon fillets, 1 cup broccoli, 1 cup sweet potatoes, olive oil, lemon slices.Instructions: Bake salmon and veggies at 400°F for 20-25 minutes, drizzle with olive oil and top with lemon slices.
2. **Zucchini Noodles with Pesto**Ingredients: 2 zucchinis, 1 cup fresh basil, 2 tbsp olive oil, garlic, lemon juice.Instructions: Spiralize zucchini into noodles. Blend basil, olive oil, garlic, and lemon juice to make pesto. Toss with zucchini noodles.

<h1 style="text-align:center">13</h1>

The Importance of Sleep, Rest and Recovery and Fitness

Rest and recovery are as essential to fitness as exercise itself. Without adequate recovery, your body cannot repair and strengthen itself effectively. This chapter will highlight the importance of rest and how to incorporate it into your routine.

When it comes to fitness, many people focus solely on exercise and nutrition, but **sleep, rest, and recovery** are just as crucial to your success. Your body needs time to repair and rebuild muscles after a workout, and this process happens primarily during rest periods, including sleep.

Sleep is essential for muscle recovery, hormone regulation, and mental clarity. During deep sleep, growth hormone levels rise, helping your muscles recover and rebuild stronger. **Rest days** give your body the break it needs to prevent overtraining, reduce the risk of injury, and allow your muscles to repair.

Without proper rest, your performance can suffer, leading to fatigue, decreased strength, and slower progress. Additionally, poor sleep and insufficient recovery can increase stress and impair your immune system, making it harder to stay on track with your fitness goals.

Incorporating enough rest and sleep into your fitness routine ensures that your body stays strong, your mind stays focused, and your progress continues smoothly!

Quality sleep is the foundation of effective recovery:

- **Muscle Repair**: During deep sleep, your body releases growth hormones that repair muscles and tissues.
- **Mental Reset**: Sleep reduces stress and improves focus, helping you stay committed to your fitness goals.
- *True-Life Example*: After struggling with sleep deprivation, Clara prioritized a bedtime routine and noticed improved performance in her workouts within weeks.

Overcoming Obstacles to Rest

Many women struggle with rest due to their busy schedules. Here's how to overcome common challenges:

- **Time Management**: Prioritize at least 7 hours of sleep by setting a consistent bedtime.
- **Digital Detox**: Turn off electronic devices an hour before bed to improve sleep quality.
- *True-Life Example*: Nina started reading before bed instead of scrolling through her phone, leading to better sleep and improved

energy.

14

Conclusion

Staying fit as a busy woman is not about perfection—it's about consistency and making small, sustainable changes. Throughout this book, you've learned how to:

- Prioritize fitness without relying on gyms.
- Incorporate simple and effective workouts into your day.
- Stay motivated, track progress, and build a routine that works.
- Understand the importance of rest and recovery.
- Importance of Sleep for Fitness
- Make fitness a natural part of your lifestyle.
- Healthy Recipes for Busy Women
- Essential Nutrients for Women

Final Words of Encouragement

You don't need hours at the gym or fancy equipment to achieve your fitness goals. Start with what you have and where you are. Celebrate every small win, and remember that consistency beats intensity over the long run.

Bonus: Resources for Continued Progress

- **Fitness Apps**: Explore apps like MyFitnessPal, Nike Training Club, or YouTube channels offering free workouts.
- **Books and Podcasts**: Read books on fitness or listen to motivational podcasts during your commute.
- **Local Groups**: Join walking or yoga groups in your area to stay active and social.

Next Steps:

- Begin with a 15-minute workout from Chapter 3.
- Join an accountability group or share your journey with a friend.
- Use the tools and strategies in this book to make fitness a lifelong habit.
- Share your success story with me. (Christiebayode@gmail.com)

Final Thought: The journey to a healthier, happier you begins now. Take the first step today—your future self will thank you.

You've got this!

If you find this book helpful for yourself, your family, or your friends, I'd greatly appreciate it if you could leave a positive review on Amazon!

Thank you.

15

Resources

8 Benefits of training at Home | Life by Daily Burn. (2022, March 1). Life by Daily Burn. https://dailyburn.com/life/fitness/8-benefits-of-training-at-home/?utm

Wigle, R. (2024b, December 19). These 4 simple tips will burn more calories — you don't even need to go to the gym. New York Post. https://nypost.com/2024/12/19/health/burn-more-calories-with-these-4-simple-tips-without-the-gym/?utm

Harvard Health. (2024, June 28). The advantages of body-weight exercise. https://www.health.harvard.edu/exercise-and-fitness/the-advantages-of-body-weight-exercise?utm

Hoyle, A. (2024b, December 26). The 30-minute kitchen workout that transformed my body. The Times. https://www.thetimes.com/life-style/health-fitness/article/30-minute-kitchen-workout-advice-anto nia-hoyle-9twg2j9ls?utm

Bauman, A. E., Reis, R. S., Sallis, J. F., Wells, J. C., Loos, R. J., & Martin, B. W. (2012). Correlates of physical activity: why are some people physically active and others not? The Lancet, 380(9838), 258–271. https://doi.org/10.1016/s0140-6736(12)60735-1

Ainsworth, B. E., Haskell, W. L., Herrmann, S. D., Meckes, N., Bassett, D. R., Tudor-Locke, C., & Leon, A. S. (2011). Compendium of physical activities: A second update of codes and MET values. Medicine and Science in Sports and Exercise, 43(8), 1575–1581. https://doi.org/10.1249/MSS.0b013e31821ece12

Wigle, R. (2024c, December 19). These 4 simple tips will burn more calories — you don't even need to go to the gym. New York Post. https://nypost.com/2024/12/19/health/burn-more-calories-with-th ese-4-simple-tips-without-the-gym/?utm

Campaigns, M. (2021, October 1). Here's How You Can Benefit from a Home Workout. The Monday Campaigns. https://www.mondaycamp aigns.org/move-it-monday/heres-how-you-can-benefit-from-a-home -workout?utm

Sarkin, J. A., Johnson, S. S., Prochaska, J. O., & Prochaska, J. M. (2001b). Applying the transtheoretical model to regular moderate exercise in an overweight population: Validation of a stages of change measure. Preventive Medicine, 33(5), 462–469. https://doi.org/10.1006/pmed.2 001.0916

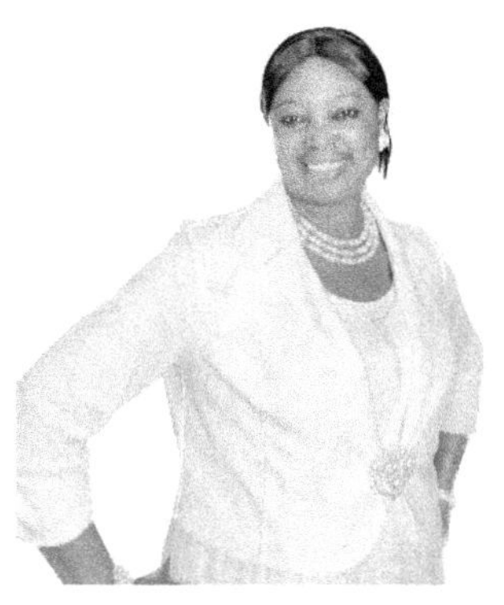

About the Author

Hi, I'm Christiana Bayode, passionate about helping busy women achieve a healthier and balanced life. My mission is to inspire women to prioritize their health and make fitness a sustainable, enjoyable part of their daily lives. I also help and assist women in starting an online Business. Please Join me on this journey to a healthier and happy lifestyle. Connect with me through my website: www.thechristiana.com to start your Online Business. Email: christiebayode@gmail.com